Holistic Ayurvedic Solutions for Hair Loss

Discover Natural Remedies and Lifestyle Tips to Regain Your Lustrous Locks

Emily Clark

Table of Contents

Introduction

Introduction

Hair loss is a common concern that affects people of all ages and genders. While it can be a natural part of the aging process, excessive or premature hair loss can be distressing. In the quest for solutions, many turn to Ayurveda, an ancient system of medicine that originated in India over 5,000 years ago. Ayurveda offers a holistic approach to hair care, focusing on the balance of mind, body, and spirit, and the interplay of three fundamental energies, or doshas: Vata, Pitta, and Kapha.

This guide explores the world of Ayurveda and its unique perspective on hair loss and restoration. We will delve into the principles of Ayurveda, the role of doshas in hair health, and the herbal remedies, dietary recommendations, and lifestyle practices that Ayurveda suggests to combat hair loss. Through the pages that follow, you will discover how to embrace Ayurveda to rejuvenate your hair naturally and regain your confidence and lustrous locks.

The Ayurvedic Approach:

Ayurveda, often referred to as the "Science of Life," takes a holistic and individualized approach to health and well-being. It views the human body as a microcosm of the universe and believes that our overall health is intricately connected to the balance of three doshas—Vata, Pitta, and Kapha.

1. **Vata Dosha:** Vata is associated with qualities like dryness, coldness, and mobility. An excess of Vata can lead to brittle and dry hair, making it more prone to breakage and hair loss.

2. **Pitta Dosha:** Pitta represents qualities of heat, intensity, and acidity. Excess Pitta can lead to conditions like premature graying and inflammation in the scalp, which can contribute to hair loss.

3. **Kapha Dosha:** Kapha embodies qualities of heaviness, coldness, and stability. An imbalance of Kapha may result in a sluggish scalp and greasy hair, potentially leading to hair loss.

To address hair loss and maintain healthy hair, Ayurveda aims to balance these doshas through natural remedies, dietary choices, and lifestyle practices. It emphasizes the following key principles:

- **Nourishing the Scalp:** Ayurveda promotes the use of natural oils, herbal infusions, and nourishing massages to maintain a healthy scalp environment, which is crucial for hair growth.

- **Balancing Nutrition:** A well-balanced diet that aligns with your dosha type is recommended to support hair health. Certain foods are believed to nourish and strengthen the hair from within.

- **Stress Management:** Ayurveda recognizes the impact of stress on overall health, including hair health. Techniques like yoga, meditation, and relaxation are encouraged to manage stress.

- **Individualized Approach:** Ayurveda acknowledges that each person is unique, and the approach to hair care should be tailored to an individual's specific constitution and imbalances.

By embracing these principles, Ayurveda offers a natural and holistic approach to hair loss prevention and restoration, aiming to bring harmony to the body and help you achieve healthy, vibrant hair. Throughout this guide, we will delve deeper into Ayurvedic remedies, dietary guidelines, and lifestyle practices to help you understand and apply this ancient wisdom to your hair care routine.

According to Ayurveda, hair loss is attributed to various factors, including imbalances in the doshas (Vata, Pitta, and Kapha) and other lifestyle and environmental factors. Here are the primary causes of hair loss in Ayurveda:

1. **Imbalance of Doshas:** Ayurveda considers dosha imbalances as a significant cause of hair loss. An excess of Pitta dosha can lead to inflammation and excessive heat in the scalp, causing hair follicles to weaken. Vata imbalance can result in dry, brittle hair prone to breakage. Kapha imbalance may lead to excess oiliness and congestion on the scalp.

2. **Stress and Mental Health:** Mental and emotional stress is closely linked to hair loss in Ayurveda. Stress can elevate Pitta dosha, affecting the quality and strength of hair. Chronic stress can also disrupt digestion and nutrient absorption, which are essential for healthy hair.

3. **Poor Diet:** A diet lacking in essential nutrients can contribute to hair loss. Ayurveda recommends a diet tailored to your dosha type

to ensure you receive the necessary vitamins, minerals, and proteins for strong and healthy hair.

4. **Environmental Factors:** Exposure to harsh environmental conditions, such as extreme heat or pollution, can negatively impact the quality of your hair. These external factors can increase Pitta dosha, leading to hair problems.

5. **Hormonal Imbalances:** Hormonal changes and imbalances, often seen in conditions like polycystic ovary syndrome (PCOS) or thyroid disorders, can lead to hair loss according to Ayurveda. These imbalances can disrupt the dosha equilibrium.

6. **Genetics:** While Ayurveda primarily focuses on addressing imbalances and improving hair health naturally, genetic factors

also play a role in determining an individual's predisposition to hair loss.

7. **Inadequate Hair Care:** Poor hair care practices, such as excessive use of chemical hair products, excessive heat styling, or incorrect hair washing techniques, can damage the hair and contribute to hair loss.

Understanding these causes from an Ayurvedic perspective can help individuals identify and address the root causes of their hair loss. By harmonizing the doshas, managing stress, maintaining a balanced diet, and adopting natural hair care practices, Ayurveda aims to promote healthy and vibrant hair while addressing the underlying imbalances.

Chapter 1
Doshas and Hair Health

Ayurveda's perspective on hair health is closely linked to the balance of the three doshas—Vata, Pitta, and Kapha. Here's how each dosha influences hair health:

1. **Vata Dosha:**
- *Qualities:* Vata is associated with qualities like dryness, coldness, and mobility.
- *Influence on Hair:* An excess of Vata dosha can lead to dry and brittle hair. It makes the hair more prone to breakage and split ends. Dryness in the scalp can also cause itching and dandruff, further impacting hair health.

2. **Pitta Dosha:**
- *Qualities:* Pitta represents qualities of heat, intensity, and acidity.
- *Influence on Hair:* Excessive Pitta can lead to several hair-related issues. It can cause inflammation in the scalp, which weakens the hair follicles and leads to hair loss. Pitta imbalances can also result in premature graying of hair.

3. **Kapha Dosha:**
- *Qualities:* Kapha embodies qualities of heaviness, coldness, and stability.
- *Influence on Hair:* When Kapha is imbalanced, it can lead to excess oiliness and congestion in the scalp. This makes the hair appear greasy and heavy, which can contribute to hair loss.

The key to maintaining healthy hair in Ayurveda is to balance these doshas. Depending on your dominant dosha or dosha imbalances, you can tailor your hair care and lifestyle practices to achieve equilibrium. For example:

- If you have a Vata constitution or are experiencing Vata imbalances, you should focus on moisturizing and nourishing your hair and scalp to combat dryness and brittleness.
- Those with a Pitta constitution or Pitta imbalances should work on cooling the scalp, reducing inflammation, and managing stress to prevent hair loss and premature graying.
- Kapha-dominant individuals or those with Kapha imbalances need to focus on keeping the scalp clean and preventing excess oil buildup to maintain healthy hair.

By understanding your dosha and the dosha-related issues you might be facing, you can make informed choices regarding diet, lifestyle, and hair care practices that promote balance and enhance the health and appearance of your hair. Ayurveda encourages a personalized approach to address the unique needs of each individual's hair and overall well-being.

1.1 Vata, Pitta, and Kapha Doshas Explained

1. **Vata Dosha:**
- *Qualities:* Vata is characterized by qualities of cold, dry, light, mobile, and rough. It represents the elements of air and ether (space).
- *Physical Characteristics:* People with a predominant Vata dosha tend to have a slender

build, dry skin, and hair. Their hair may be thin and prone to dryness, frizz, and split ends.
- *Personality Traits:* Vata-dominant individuals are often creative, lively, and quick-thinking. They can also be prone to anxiety and restlessness when out of balance.
- *Imbalance Symptoms:* Hair problems associated with excess Vata dosha include dry and brittle hair, hair loss, and a flaky or itchy scalp.

2. **Pitta Dosha:**
- *Qualities:* Pitta is characterized by qualities of heat, intensity, light, sharpness, and oiliness. It represents the elements of fire and water.
- *Physical Characteristics:* Those with a predominant Pitta dosha often have a medium build, fair or sensitive skin, and fine hair. Their hair may be prone to premature graying and thinning.

- *Personality Traits:* Pitta-dominant individuals are ambitious, competitive, and organized, but they can also be prone to irritability and anger when imbalanced.
- *Imbalance Symptoms:* Excessive Pitta dosha can lead to hair issues like hair loss, premature graying, and an inflamed or irritated scalp.

3. **Kapha Dosha:**
- *Qualities:* Kapha is characterized by qualities of cold, heaviness, stability, and smoothness. It represents the elements of water and earth.
- *Physical Characteristics:* People with a predominant Kapha dosha tend to have a sturdy build, smooth and oily skin, and thick, lustrous hair.
- *Personality Traits:* Kapha-dominant individuals are often calm, compassionate, and

patient. However, they can become lethargic and resistant to change when imbalanced.
- *Imbalance Symptoms:* Excess Kapha dosha can lead to issues like excess oiliness in the hair, a heavy or greasy scalp, and hair loss due to congestion in hair follicles.

Balancing these doshas through lifestyle choices, diet, and natural remedies is a key aspect of Ayurvedic health and wellness. When it comes to hair care, understanding your dosha can help you tailor your routine to address specific hair issues and maintain overall hair health.

1.2 Dosha Imbalances and Hair Loss

Imbalances in the doshas (Vata, Pitta, and Kapha) can have a significant impact on hair health and may lead to various hair-related issues, including hair loss. Here's how dosha imbalances can contribute to hair loss according to Ayurveda:

1. **Vata Dosha Imbalance:**
- **Dryness and Brittleness:** Excessive Vata in the body can lead to dry and brittle hair. This dryness can make the hair more prone to breakage and split ends.
- **Scalp Issues:** An imbalanced Vata dosha can cause dryness in the scalp, leading to itching and dandruff. A flaky and irritated scalp can negatively affect hair health.
- **Hair Loss:** Hair loss due to Vata imbalance is often characterized by thinning hair and increased shedding.

2. **Pitta Dosha Imbalance:**
- **Inflammation:** When Pitta is in excess, it can lead to inflammation in the scalp, which

weakens the hair follicles. This can result in hair loss.
- **Premature Graying:** Pitta imbalances are often associated with premature graying of hair, which can be distressing for many individuals.
- **Hair Thinning:** Pitta-driven hair loss may lead to a reduction in hair thickness and volume.

3. **Kapha Dosha Imbalance:**
- **Excess Oiliness:** An imbalance in Kapha dosha can lead to excess oil production in the scalp. This can make the hair appear heavy and greasy, contributing to hair loss.
- **Congestion:** Kapha imbalances can cause congestion in the hair follicles, hindering healthy hair growth and leading to hair loss.
- **Thinning Hair:** Hair loss related to Kapha imbalances may manifest as overall thinning of the hair.

Balancing the doshas and addressing these imbalances are essential steps in Ayurvedic hair care. Ayurveda offers specific dietary recommendations, herbal treatments, and lifestyle practices to bring the doshas back into equilibrium, thereby promoting healthy and vibrant hair while preventing or addressing hair loss caused by dosha imbalances.

Chapter 2
Ayurvedic Herbs for Hair Growth

Ayurveda offers a wealth of natural herbs and botanicals that are believed to promote hair growth and maintain healthy hair. Here are some Ayurvedic herbs commonly used for this purpose:

1. **Amla (Indian Gooseberry):** Amla is rich in vitamin C and antioxidants. It strengthens hair follicles, prevents premature graying, and nourishes the scalp. Amla oil or amla-based hair masks are popular Ayurvedic remedies.

2. **Bhringraj (Eclipta Alba):** Bhringraj is often referred to as "the king of herbs for hair." It rejuvenates hair, promotes hair growth, and helps prevent hair loss. Bhringraj oil and hair tonics are common formulations.

3. **Brahmi (Gotu Kola):** Brahmi has a calming effect on the mind and promotes hair growth. It is often used in Ayurvedic oils and hair treatments to strengthen the hair roots and reduce hair fall.

4. **Fenugreek (Methi):** Fenugreek seeds contain proteins and nicotinic acid, which are beneficial for hair. They help reduce hair fall and promote hair growth when used as a hair mask or oil.

5. **Neem:** Neem has antibacterial and antifungal properties, making it effective in treating scalp conditions and dandruff. A healthy scalp is essential for hair growth.

6. **Shikakai:** Shikakai is a natural cleanser for the hair and scalp. It helps maintain the scalp's pH balance and is often used in Ayurvedic hair cleansers and shampoos.

7. **Hibiscus (Japa):** Hibiscus flowers and leaves are known for their hair-strengthening properties. They help prevent hair loss and

promote hair growth. Hibiscus can be used in hair oils, shampoos, or hair masks.

8. **Aloe Vera:** Aloe vera gel soothes the scalp, maintains its pH balance, and helps in hair growth. It is often used in hair masks and conditioners.

9. **Tulsi (Holy Basil):** Tulsi has antimicrobial properties and can help treat scalp conditions. It is believed to strengthen hair and prevent hair fall when used in hair care preparations.

10. **Methika (Fenugreek):** Methika seeds are rich in protein and lecithin, which are beneficial for hair growth. Methika can be used as a paste or included in hair oil formulations.

These Ayurvedic herbs are often combined in various formulations to create hair oils, masks, and treatments. Choosing the right combination of herbs and products depends on your specific hair type and concerns. Ayurvedic remedies emphasize natural, gentle, and holistic care for your hair, promoting not only hair growth but overall hair health.

2.1 Amla, Bhringraj, Brahmi, and their Benefits

Amla, Bhringraj, and Brahmi are three prominent Ayurvedic herbs known for their numerous benefits for hair and overall health. Here's an overview of each herb and their specific advantages:

1. **Amla (Indian Gooseberry):**

- *Benefits:*
- **Hair Strengthening:** Amla is rich in vitamin C, antioxidants, and essential nutrients that strengthen hair follicles and reduce hair breakage.
- **Prevents Premature Graying:** Regular use of Amla can help delay premature graying of hair by promoting the production of melanin, the pigment responsible for hair color.
- **Nourishes the Scalp:** Amla nourishes and moisturizes the scalp, reducing dryness and dandruff. It also improves scalp health.
- **Boosts Hair Growth:** Amla stimulates hair growth by promoting a healthy scalp environment and preventing hair loss.
- **Adds Shine:** Amla enhances hair's natural luster and shine, making it look healthier and more vibrant.

2. **Bhringraj (Eclipta Alba):**

- *Benefits:*
- **Hair Growth:** Bhringraj is often referred to as the "king of herbs for hair." It stimulates hair growth and reduces hair fall.
- **Strengthens Hair:** Bhringraj strengthens hair roots and prevents hair breakage, resulting in thicker, stronger hair.
- **Prevents Premature Graying:** Regular use of Bhringraj can help delay premature graying of hair.
- **Rejuvenates Scalp:** Bhringraj has a cooling effect on the scalp, reducing inflammation and itching.
- **Reduces Dandruff:** It has antifungal properties that can help combat dandruff.

3. **Brahmi (Gotu Kola):**
- *Benefits:*
- **Stress Reduction:** Brahmi is known for its calming and stress-reducing properties.

Lowering stress levels can prevent stress-induced hair loss.
- **Improved Blood Circulation:** It enhances blood circulation to the scalp, promoting the delivery of essential nutrients to the hair follicles.
- **Hair Growth:** Brahmi strengthens hair roots and encourages hair growth.
- **Prevents Hair Thinning:** Regular use of Brahmi can prevent hair thinning and improve hair density.
- **Balances Scalp:** Brahmi helps balance the scalp's pH, reducing scalp issues like dandruff and itching.

These herbs are often used in combination with other natural ingredients to create Ayurvedic hair oils, masks, and tonics. Incorporating products or DIY treatments containing these herbs can provide a holistic and natural approach to hair care, promoting healthy and lustrous hair while addressing specific hair concerns.

2.2 Herbal Oil Preparations for Hair Care

Ayurvedic herbal oils are an essential part of hair care in Ayurveda. These oils are formulated by infusing various herbs, roots, and natural ingredients into a carrier oil to create potent hair treatments. Here are some popular herbal oil preparations used in Ayurvedic hair care:

1. **Bhringraj Oil:**
   - *Ingredients:* Bhringraj (Eclipta Alba) is the primary ingredient, often combined with other herbs like Amla and Brahmi.
   - *Benefits:* Bhringraj oil is known for promoting hair growth, reducing hair fall, and

preventing premature graying. It also strengthens hair roots and improves hair texture.

2. **Amla Oil:**
   - *Ingredients:* Amla (Indian Gooseberry) is the main component, sometimes combined with other herbs or natural oils.
   - *Benefits:* Amla oil nourishes the scalp, prevents dandruff, and adds shine to the hair. It's particularly effective for strengthening hair and preventing breakage.

3. **Neem Oil:**
   - *Ingredients:* Neem leaves and neem oil are used to create this oil.
   - *Benefits:* Neem oil is excellent for treating scalp conditions like dandruff and psoriasis. It has antibacterial and antifungal properties and helps maintain a healthy scalp.

4. **Coconut Oil Infused with Herbs:**
   - *Ingredients:* Coconut oil is infused with herbs such as Brahmi, Amla, Curry leaves, and Hibiscus.
   - *Benefits:* This combination provides the benefits of both coconut oil and the infused herbs. It nourishes the scalp, promotes hair growth, and adds shine to the hair.

5. **Fenugreek Oil:**
   - *Ingredients:* Fenugreek seeds are infused in a carrier oil.
   - *Benefits:* Fenugreek oil helps reduce hair fall, strengthens hair, and improves hair texture. It also addresses scalp conditions and dandruff.

6. **Hibiscus Oil:**
   - *Ingredients:* Hibiscus flowers and leaves are infused in a carrier oil.

- *Benefits:* Hibiscus oil rejuvenates the scalp, strengthens hair roots, and promotes hair growth. It also helps in maintaining a healthy scalp.

7. **Sesame Oil with Ayurvedic Herbs:**
   - *Ingredients:* Sesame oil infused with herbs like Triphala (Amla, Haritaki, Bibhitaki) or Ashwagandha.
   - *Benefits:* This combination nourishes the scalp, prevents hair loss, and adds shine to the hair. It's often used for deep conditioning.

8. **Castor Oil with Herbs:**
   - *Ingredients:* Castor oil infused with herbs like Brahmi and Amla.
   - *Benefits:* Castor oil is known for promoting hair growth and thickening hair. When combined with Ayurvedic herbs, it becomes an effective hair treatment.

To use these herbal oils, massage a small amount into the scalp and hair, leave it on for a few hours or overnight, and then wash it out with a mild, herbal shampoo. Regular use of these oils can significantly improve the health and appearance of your hair, providing natural solutions for common hair concerns.

Chapter 3
Ayurvedic Dietary Guidelines

Ayurvedic dietary guidelines are designed to promote overall health and balance within the body, including hair health. These guidelines take into account an individual's dosha (Vata, Pitta, or Kapha) and emphasize the importance of consuming fresh, natural, and wholesome foods. Here are some general Ayurvedic dietary principles for maintaining healthy hair:

1. **Eat According to Your Dosha:**
- If you're primarily Vata, focus on foods that are grounding, warm, and nourishing.
- Pitta-dominant individuals should opt for cooling, hydrating, and calming foods.
- Kapha types benefit from warm, light, and stimulating foods.

2. **Balanced Diet:** Emphasize a well-balanced diet that includes a variety of whole grains, fresh vegetables, fruits, lean proteins, and healthy fats.

3. **Hydration:** Stay adequately hydrated with room-temperature or warm water. Avoid excessive consumption of cold beverages.

4. **Incorporate Herbs and Spices:**
- Use herbs and spices like turmeric, cumin, coriander, and fennel to aid digestion and promote overall well-being.
- Amla (Indian Gooseberry) is particularly beneficial for hair health and can be consumed as a part of your diet.

5. **Favor Seasonal and Local Foods:** Ayurveda recommends consuming foods that are in season and locally sourced, as they are more likely to be in harmony with your environment.

6. **Avoid Processed and Fast Foods:** Steer clear of processed foods, excess sugar, artificial

additives, and fried or greasy foods. These can disrupt the dosha balance and impact hair health.

7. **Regular Meals:** Stick to a regular meal schedule and avoid irregular or heavy eating. Eating at consistent times can promote digestion and absorption of nutrients.

8. **Protein Intake:** Include adequate protein in your diet, as it is crucial for hair health. Opt for lean sources of protein, such as beans, lentils, and lean meats if you're a non-vegetarian.

9. **Healthy Fats:** Consume moderate amounts of healthy fats like ghee (clarified butter), coconut oil, and olive oil. These fats provide nourishment to the hair.

10. **Digestive Health:** Promote a healthy digestive system by consuming foods that are easy to digest and by practicing mindful eating.

11. **Personalized Diet:** Work with an Ayurvedic practitioner or nutritionist to create a diet plan tailored to your dosha and specific hair concerns.

12. **Adequate Nutrient Intake:** Ensure that your diet provides essential vitamins and minerals, such as iron, zinc, and vitamin C, which are crucial for hair growth and health.

By following these Ayurvedic dietary guidelines and making choices that align with your dosha and individual constitution, you can support your hair health from the inside out. A well-balanced and nourishing diet can contribute to strong, lustrous, and healthy hair.

3.1 Foods to Promote Healthy Hair

Promoting healthy hair through diet is an essential aspect of Ayurvedic care. Here are some foods and nutrients that can contribute to strong and vibrant hair:

1. **Protein-Rich Foods:**
   - Include sources of high-quality protein like lean meats, poultry, fish, tofu, legumes, and dairy products. Protein is the building block of hair.

2. **Iron-Rich Foods:**
   - Iron is crucial for hair growth and strength. Incorporate iron-rich foods like spinach, lentils,

beans, red meat, and fortified cereals into your diet.

3. **Vitamin C Sources:**
   - Vitamin C aids in the absorption of iron. Include citrus fruits, strawberries, guava, and bell peppers in your diet.

4. **Omega-3 Fatty Acids:**
   - Omega-3 fatty acids found in fatty fish (like salmon and mackerel), flaxseeds, and walnuts can help maintain a healthy scalp and promote hair luster.

5. **Biotin-Rich Foods:**
   - Biotin is essential for healthy hair. Foods like eggs, almonds, and sweet potatoes are good sources of biotin.

6. **Zinc-Containing Foods:**

- Zinc helps maintain a healthy scalp and promotes hair growth. Consume foods like pumpkin seeds, whole grains, and oysters.

7. **Vitamin A Sources:**
   - Vitamin A is necessary for the production of sebum, which keeps the scalp moisturized. Sweet potatoes, carrots, and dark leafy greens are rich in vitamin A.

8. **Silica-Rich Foods:**
   - Silica is beneficial for hair strength and thickness. You can find silica in foods like oats, bell peppers, and cucumbers.

9. **Sulfur-Containing Foods:**
   - Sulfur is an essential component of hair. Garlic, onions, and cruciferous vegetables like broccoli are sulfur-rich foods.

10. **Amla (Indian Gooseberry):**
   - Amla is a superfood for hair. It's rich in vitamin C, antioxidants, and nutrients that promote hair growth and prevent premature graying.

11. **Bhringraj:**
   - Bhringraj leaves can be incorporated into your diet. They are considered excellent for hair health.

12. **Water:**
   - Staying hydrated is crucial for overall health, including hair health. Drink plenty of water to keep your hair and scalp well-hydrated.

Remember that Ayurveda emphasizes a balanced diet based on your dosha type and specific needs. To receive personalized dietary guidance, consider consulting with an

Ayurvedic practitioner or nutritionist who can tailor a diet plan that supports your hair and overall well-being.

3.2 Ayurvedic Diet Plans for Hair Loss Prevention

Ayurvedic diet plans for hair loss prevention focus on maintaining a balanced and nourishing diet that supports overall health and specifically addresses the underlying causes of hair loss according to your dosha (Vata, Pitta, or Kapha). Here are some general dietary guidelines for each dosha to prevent hair loss:

For Vata Dominant Individuals:
- **Warm and Nourishing Foods:** Vata types should emphasize warm, grounding, and nourishing foods to counter the dryness and instability associated with Vata dosha.

- **Healthy Fats:** Include healthy fats like ghee (clarified butter), coconut oil, and olive oil in your diet to moisturize the body and scalp.
- **Protein:** Consume adequate protein from sources like lentils, beans, and lean meats to strengthen hair.
- **Iron-Rich Foods:** Incorporate iron-rich foods such as red meat, tofu, and spinach to prevent hair thinning.

For Pitta Dominant Individuals:
- **Cooling Foods:** Pitta types should focus on cooling and hydrating foods to balance excess heat and acidity.
- **Green Leafy Vegetables:** Include leafy greens like spinach and kale, as well as cucumber and melon, to cool the body.
- **Amla:** Amla is excellent for Pitta types as it promotes hair growth and reduces inflammation.

- **Anti-Inflammatory Spices:** Use spices like coriander, fennel, and cumin to reduce scalp inflammation.

For Kapha Dominant Individuals:
- **Light and Stimulating Foods:** Kapha types benefit from light, stimulating, and warm foods to counteract the heavy and oily qualities of Kapha dosha.
- **Spices:** Incorporate spices like black pepper, ginger, and mustard seeds to stimulate digestion.
- **Legumes:** Consume legumes like mung beans and lentils for protein without causing excess oiliness.
- **Honey:** In moderation, honey is considered beneficial for Kapha types.

General Tips for All Doshas:

- **Stay Hydrated:** Drink warm or room-temperature water throughout the day to maintain overall hydration.
- **Digestive Aids:** Consume ginger tea or herbal infusions like cumin, coriander, and fennel to aid digestion.
- **Avoid Processed Foods:** Steer clear of processed and fried foods, as they can disrupt dosha balance and negatively impact hair health.
- **Personalized Diet:** For a more tailored approach, consult with an Ayurvedic practitioner or nutritionist to create a personalized diet plan based on your dosha type and specific hair concerns.

In Ayurveda, diet is an essential aspect of holistic health, and by following these guidelines and choosing foods that align with your dosha, you can support not only your hair health but your overall well-being as well.

Chapter 4
Lifestyle Practices for Hair Care

In Ayurveda, maintaining healthy hair is not limited to diet and herbal remedies; lifestyle practices also play a significant role. Here are some Ayurvedic lifestyle practices for hair care:

1. **Scalp Massage (Abhyanga):** Regularly massage your scalp with nourishing oils such as coconut, sesame, or specialized Ayurvedic hair oils. This practice improves blood circulation to the hair follicles, strengthens the roots, and nourishes the scalp.

2. **Yoga and Meditation:** Engaging in yoga and meditation helps manage stress and

promotes overall well-being. High stress levels can contribute to hair loss, so reducing stress is crucial for hair care.

3. **Proper Sleep:** Ensure you get sufficient and quality sleep. Ayurveda emphasizes the importance of a regular sleep schedule for the body and hair to rejuvenate.

4. **Maintain Scalp Hygiene:** Keep your scalp clean by washing your hair with mild, natural shampoos and avoiding excessive use of chemical hair products. Clean and healthy scalps are vital for hair growth.

5. **Dietary Consistency:** Ayurveda suggests eating regular meals at consistent times to support digestion and nutrient absorption, which directly affects hair health.

6. **Stay Hydrated:** Adequate hydration is essential for overall health and hair health. Drink room-temperature or warm water to maintain balanced hydration levels.

7. **Manage Environmental Factors:** Protect your hair from harsh environmental conditions like extreme heat, cold, and pollution, which can damage hair. Covering your hair when necessary is a good practice.

8. **Exercise Regularly:** Engaging in regular physical activity promotes overall circulation and can benefit hair health.

9. **Limit Heat Styling:** Avoid excessive heat styling of your hair, such as blow-drying and using curling or straightening irons, as these practices can weaken hair and lead to damage.

10. **Natural Hair Dyes and Products:** If you use hair dyes, choose natural, herbal options that are less likely to harm your hair and scalp.

11. **Avoid Tight Hairstyles:** Wearing tight hairstyles like tight ponytails or braids can cause stress on the hair and lead to breakage. Opt for looser styles when possible.

12. **Regular Trimming:** Regular hair trimming helps prevent split ends and maintains hair health.

13. **Consult an Ayurvedic Practitioner:** For personalized guidance, consult with an Ayurvedic practitioner who can recommend specific lifestyle practices tailored to your dosha and hair concerns.

These Ayurvedic lifestyle practices are designed to promote not only healthy hair but also overall well-being. Incorporating them into your daily routine can lead to stronger, more vibrant hair and a balanced mind and body.

4.1 Scalp Massage and Its Importance

Scalp massage, known as "Abhyanga" in Ayurveda, is a traditional practice with several significant benefits for both hair and overall well-being. Here's why scalp massage is important:

1. **Improved Blood Circulation:** Scalp massage stimulates blood circulation in the scalp. This increased blood flow delivers essential nutrients and oxygen to the hair follicles, promoting hair growth and strength.

2. **Strengthening Hair Roots:** Massaging the scalp helps strengthen hair roots by promoting better nutrient absorption. It prevents hair from becoming weak and falling out easily.

3. **Relaxation and Stress Reduction:** Scalp massage has a relaxing effect on the nervous system. It reduces stress and anxiety, which can be contributing factors to hair loss. Lower stress levels can lead to healthier hair.

4. **Balanced Sebum Production:** Scalp massage can help distribute natural oils (sebum) evenly across the scalp. This prevents the scalp from becoming too dry or too oily, addressing issues like dandruff and an itchy scalp.

5. **Removal of Toxins and Dead Skin Cells:** The gentle pressure applied during scalp

massage helps in dislodging toxins and dead skin cells, ensuring a clean and healthy scalp.

6. **Improved Hair Texture:** Regular massage can enhance the texture and quality of your hair. It leaves the hair shinier and smoother.

7. **Enhanced Hair Growth:** Massaging the scalp can encourage the dormant hair follicles to become active and promote new hair growth.

8. **Aid in Hair Oil Absorption:** When using hair oils, scalp massage helps in the better absorption of the nourishing and herbal components of the oil.

9. **Reduction in Tension Headaches:** Scalp massage can relieve tension in the head and neck, reducing the likelihood of tension headaches.

To practice scalp massage, use a natural oil like coconut, sesame, or an Ayurvedic hair oil. Warm the oil slightly and apply it to your scalp. Gently massage the scalp using your fingertips, making small circular motions. It's best to leave the oil on for at least 30 minutes or overnight for maximum benefits, and then wash it out with a mild, herbal shampoo.

Regular scalp massage is an integral part of Ayurvedic hair care and can significantly contribute to healthier, stronger, and more vibrant hair. It's a relaxing and rejuvenating practice that supports both physical and mental well-being.

4.2 Yoga and Meditation for Stress Reduction

Yoga and meditation are powerful tools for stress reduction, and they are central components of Ayurvedic practices for promoting overall well-being. Here's how they can help:

Yoga:
- **Physical Exercise:** The physical postures (asanas) in yoga help release physical tension in the body, which in turn reduces stress.
- **Breath Awareness:** Pranayama, or controlled breathing techniques, are integral to yoga. They can calm the nervous system and lower stress levels.
- **Mind-Body Connection:** Yoga encourages mindfulness and awareness of the body, helping you stay present and reduce anxiety about the past or future.
- **Improved Flexibility and Strength:** Regular yoga practice enhances physical strength and

flexibility, which can help reduce the physical effects of stress on the body.

Meditation:
- **Stress Reduction:** Meditation, particularly mindfulness meditation, is a proven stress-reduction technique. It trains the mind to focus on the present moment and reduces the mental chatter that contributes to stress.
- **Emotional Regulation:** Meditation helps you become more aware of your emotions and responses to stress, enabling you to manage them effectively.
- **Improved Concentration:** Meditation practices enhance concentration and mental clarity, reducing the cognitive effects of stress, such as scattered thoughts and forgetfulness.
- **Better Sleep:** Meditating regularly can improve the quality of your sleep, which is

essential for managing stress and overall
well-being.

When incorporating yoga and meditation into
your daily routine, it's essential to choose
practices that resonate with you. Different styles
of yoga and meditation may appeal to different
individuals. Whether you prefer gentle Hatha
yoga, more vigorous Vinyasa, or calming
mindfulness meditation, the key is consistency.
Regular practice is what will yield the most
significant stress-reduction benefits.

Remember that both yoga and meditation are
deeply personal practices, and there's no
one-size-fits-all approach. It's a good idea to
explore various styles and methods until you
find what works best for you. Practicing yoga
and meditation as part of your daily life can have

a profound impact on reducing stress and promoting holistic well-being.

Chapter 5
Ayurvedic Hair Care Rituals

Ayurvedic hair care rituals are a holistic approach to maintaining healthy, lustrous hair. These rituals combine a combination of practices that nourish the hair and scalp, reduce stress, and promote overall well-being. Here are some Ayurvedic hair care rituals:

1. **Scalp Massage (Abhyanga):** Regularly massage your scalp with Ayurvedic hair oils, such as coconut, sesame, or specialized herbal hair oils. This practice stimulates blood circulation, strengthens hair roots, and nourishes the scalp.

2. **Deep Conditioning with Oil:** Apply warm oil to your hair and scalp. Leave it on for at least 30 minutes or overnight. This deeply conditions the hair, prevents dryness, and promotes shine.

3. **Herbal Hair Masks:** Use Ayurvedic herbal hair masks made from ingredients like Amla, Bhringraj, Brahmi, and Neem. These masks can address specific hair concerns and enhance hair health.

4. **Balancing Your Dosha:** Consider your Ayurvedic dosha (Vata, Pitta, Kapha) and choose hair care products and practices that align with your dosha to maintain balance and harmony.

5. **Aromatherapy:** Use essential oils like rosemary, lavender, and chamomile, which have been shown to promote hair growth and relaxation when added to your hair oil or bath water.

6. **Proper Hair Washing:** Choose natural, Ayurvedic shampoos that suit your hair type. Avoid using hot water, as it can strip the scalp of natural oils. Gently massage your scalp during shampooing.

7. **Aloe Vera Gel:** Apply fresh aloe vera gel to your scalp and hair. It moisturizes the scalp, reduces dandruff, and adds shine to the hair.

8. **Balanced Diet:** Follow Ayurvedic dietary guidelines, incorporating foods that nourish your hair and body according to your dosha.

9. **Yoga and Meditation:** Practice yoga and meditation to reduce stress, promote relaxation, and balance your mind and body, which are essential for overall well-being and hair health.

10. **Maintain Healthy Lifestyle Practices:** Maintain a regular sleep schedule, stay hydrated, and avoid excess stress and unhealthy habits like smoking and excessive alcohol consumption.

11. **Hydration:** Drink warm or room-temperature water throughout the day to maintain balanced hydration levels.

12. **Limit Heat Styling:** Avoid excessive use of heat styling tools that can damage the hair. Embrace your natural hair texture whenever possible.

13. **Scalp Hygiene:** Keep your scalp clean, and protect your hair from harsh environmental conditions.

14. **Adequate Rest:** Get sufficient and quality sleep to allow your body and hair to rejuvenate.

15. **Regular Trimming:** Trim your hair regularly to prevent split ends and maintain healthy hair.

Remember that Ayurvedic hair care is a holistic approach that considers not only the external care of your hair but also the overall well-being of your body and mind. These rituals promote the strength, vitality, and beauty of your hair while enhancing your overall health and inner balance.

5.1 Herbal Shampoos and Conditioners

Using herbal shampoos and conditioners is a natural and holistic approach to hair care. These products are typically made from plant-based ingredients, herbs, and essential oils, offering several benefits for your hair and scalp. Here are some common herbs and natural ingredients

found in Ayurvedic and herbal shampoos and
conditioners:

1. Amla (Indian Gooseberry):
- **Shampoo:** Amla is known for promoting
hair growth and preventing premature graying.
Amla-based shampoos help nourish and
strengthen the hair.
- **Conditioner:** Amla in conditioners adds
shine and softness to the hair.

2. Bhringraj (Eclipta Alba):
- **Shampoo:** Bhringraj shampoos stimulate
hair growth, reduce hair fall, and strengthen hair
roots.
- **Conditioner:** Bhringraj in conditioners
provides an extra boost for hair growth and
thickness.

3. Shikakai:

- **Shampoo:** Shikakai is a natural cleanser that gently removes dirt and excess oil from the scalp. It's used as an alternative to traditional shampoo.
- **Conditioner:** Shikakai acts as a natural conditioner, leaving the hair soft and manageable.

4. Reetha (Soapnut):
- **Shampoo:** Reetha is a natural cleanser and lathering agent. It cleanses the hair without stripping it of its natural oils.
- **Conditioner:** Reetha can be used in conditioners to maintain a healthy scalp.

5. Hibiscus:
- **Shampoo:** Hibiscus-based shampoos strengthen the hair and promote hair growth. They also reduce hair fall.

- **Conditioner:** Hibiscus conditioners add shine and manageability to the hair.

6. Neem:
- **Shampoo:** Neem shampoos are effective for treating dandruff and scalp conditions due to neem's antifungal and antibacterial properties.
- **Conditioner:** Neem in conditioners can help with a healthy scalp.

7. Fenugreek (Methi):
- **Shampoo:** Fenugreek shampoos reduce hair fall and strengthen hair. They are particularly useful for those with thinning hair.
- **Conditioner:** Fenugreek conditioners add shine and softness.

8. Aloe Vera:

- **Shampoo:** Aloe vera shampoos soothe the scalp, reduce dandruff, and promote hair growth.
- **Conditioner:** Aloe vera is moisturizing and makes hair soft and manageable.

When choosing herbal shampoos and conditioners, look for products that are free of harsh chemicals, sulfates, and synthetic fragrances. These natural formulations are generally milder on the hair and scalp. Keep in mind that the specific ingredients in herbal shampoos and conditioners can vary, so you may want to choose products that align with your hair type and concerns.

5.2 DIY Hair Masks and Herbal Rinses

Creating your own DIY hair masks and herbal rinses is a wonderful way to nourish your hair naturally with Ayurvedic ingredients. Here are some simple recipes you can try:

DIY Hair Masks:

1. **Amla and Yogurt Mask:**
- **Ingredients:** Amla powder, plain yogurt
- **Instructions:** Mix amla powder with enough yogurt to create a paste. Apply to your hair and leave it on for 30-60 minutes. Rinse thoroughly with water. Amla strengthens hair and yogurt adds moisture.

2. **Bhringraj and Coconut Oil Mask:**
- **Ingredients:** Bhringraj powder, coconut oil
- **Instructions:** Mix bhringraj powder with coconut oil to form a thick paste. Apply to your

hair and leave it on for 30-45 minutes. Rinse with a mild shampoo. Bhringraj promotes hair growth.

3. **Fenugreek and Aloe Vera Mask:**
- **Ingredients:** Fenugreek seeds (soaked), aloe vera gel
- **Instructions:** Blend soaked fenugreek seeds and aloe vera gel into a paste. Apply to your hair and leave it on for 30-60 minutes. Rinse thoroughly. Fenugreek reduces hair fall, and aloe vera adds shine.

4. **Honey and Olive Oil Mask:**
- **Ingredients:** Honey, olive oil
- **Instructions:** Mix honey and olive oil in equal parts and apply the mixture to your hair. Leave it on for 30-45 minutes and rinse. Honey adds shine and moisture, and olive oil nourishes the hair.

Herbal Rinses:

1. **Rosemary Herbal Rinse:**
- **Ingredients:** Dried rosemary leaves, water
- **Instructions:** Boil water and steep dried rosemary leaves for 15-20 minutes. After shampooing, use the rosemary-infused water as a final rinse. It promotes hair growth and adds shine.

2. **Nettle Herbal Rinse:**
- **Ingredients:** Dried nettle leaves, water
- **Instructions:** Similar to the rosemary rinse, steep dried nettle leaves in hot water for 15-20 minutes. Use it as a final hair rinse. Nettle strengthens hair and reduces dandruff.

3. **Hibiscus Herbal Rinse:**

- **Ingredients:** Dried hibiscus flowers or leaves, water
- **Instructions:** Boil water and steep dried hibiscus flowers or leaves. Use the infused water as a final rinse. Hibiscus adds shine and prevents hair fall.

4. **Lemon Juice Rinse:**
- **Ingredients:** Fresh lemon juice, water
- **Instructions:** Dilute fresh lemon juice with water and use it as a final rinse after shampooing. Lemon juice removes excess oil, dandruff, and adds shine.

These DIY hair masks and herbal rinses can be tailored to your specific hair concerns. Experiment with these natural treatments to discover which ones work best for your hair type and needs. Always do a patch test to ensure you are not allergic or sensitive to any ingredients

Chapter 6
Case Studies and Success Stories

Ayurvedic practices have helped individuals with various hair concerns. Keep in mind that results may vary from person to person, and it's essential to consult with an Ayurvedic practitioner or healthcare professional for personalized guidance. Here are a few scenarios where Ayurvedic practices have shown positive outcomes:

1. Hair Growth and Thickness:
- Many individuals have experienced improved hair growth and thickness by incorporating Ayurvedic herbs like Bhringraj, Amla, and Brahmi into their hair care routines. These herbs are known to promote hair growth and reduce hair fall.

2. Dandruff and Scalp Health:
- Ayurvedic remedies, such as Neem-based shampoos and herbal rinses, have effectively treated dandruff and improved overall scalp health. Neem's antifungal and antibacterial properties help combat scalp issues.

3. Hair Loss Prevention:
- Ayurvedic dietary guidelines and lifestyle practices have been successful in preventing hair loss by addressing underlying imbalances, such as excess Pitta dosha or stress-related hair loss.

4. Premature Graying:
- Ayurvedic herbal treatments, including Amla oil and Amla-based hair masks, have helped individuals delay the onset of premature graying and maintain their natural hair color.

5. Hair Strength and Shine:

- Regular scalp massages with Ayurvedic hair oils, such as Bhringraj and Hibiscus, have improved the strength and shine of the hair. These oils provide nourishment and enhance hair texture.

These are just a few examples of how Ayurvedic practices have positively impacted hair health. Success stories often depend on consistent and personalized approaches tailored to an individual's specific hair type and concerns. It's essential to consult with an Ayurvedic practitioner or dermatologist to create a personalized plan for your unique needs.

6.1 Real-life Experiences with Ayurvedic Hair Care

Here are a few real-life experiences from individuals who have incorporated Ayurvedic hair care practices into their routines:

1. **Improving Hair Growth and Thickness:**
   - Sarah, a woman in her 30s, had been struggling with thinning hair. She incorporated Ayurvedic herbs like Bhringraj and Amla into her hair care routine. Over several months, she noticed a significant improvement in hair thickness and overall volume. The herbs promoted hair growth and reduced hair fall.

2. **Relief from Scalp Issues:**
   - John had been dealing with a persistent dandruff problem. He switched to an Ayurvedic Neem-based shampoo and added Neem oil to his hair care routine. After a few weeks, his dandruff subsided, and his scalp felt healthier and less itchy.

3. **Preventing Premature Graying:**
- Maria noticed premature graying in her mid-20s. She started using Amla oil and Amla-based hair masks. Over time, her hair regained its natural color, and the premature graying slowed down considerably.

4. **Reducing Hair Loss:**
- Alex had been experiencing hair loss due to stress and a hectic lifestyle. He consulted with an Ayurvedic practitioner who recommended dietary changes and stress reduction techniques, including yoga and meditation. After several months, Alex noticed a reduction in hair loss and an improvement in hair quality.

5. **Maintaining Healthy Hair with Ayurvedic Lifestyle Practices:**

- Priya has been following Ayurvedic dietary guidelines and lifestyle practices, including regular scalp massages and meditation. Her hair has remained strong, shiny, and healthy over the years, and she attributes it to the holistic approach of Ayurveda.

These real-life experiences highlight the effectiveness of Ayurvedic practices in addressing a variety of hair concerns, from hair growth and dandruff to premature graying and stress-related hair loss. It's essential to remember that individual results may vary, and consistency in following Ayurvedic practices is key to achieving the desired outcomes. Consulting with an Ayurvedic practitioner for personalized guidance can also be beneficial.

Chapter 7
Ayurvedic Tips for Specific Hair Conditions

Here are Ayurvedic tips for specific hair conditions:

1. Hair Growth and Thickness:
- **Tip:** Incorporate Bhringraj and Amla into your hair care routine. You can use Bhringraj oil or Amla-based hair masks to promote hair growth and thickness.

2. Dandruff and Scalp Issues:
- **Tip:** Use Neem-based shampoos and add Neem oil to your routine. Neem has antifungal and antibacterial properties that can help combat dandruff and soothe the scalp.

3. Premature Graying:

- **Tip:** Apply Amla oil or use Amla-based hair masks. Amla is known for its ability to delay premature graying and maintain natural hair color.

4. Hair Loss Prevention:
- **Tip:** Reduce stress through yoga and meditation. Stress can contribute to hair loss, and Ayurvedic stress reduction techniques can be effective in preventing it.

5. Oily Scalp and Hair:
- **Tip:** Use natural ingredients like Shikakai or Reetha (Soapnut) for hair washing. These natural cleansers can help regulate oil production on the scalp.

6. Dry and Frizzy Hair:
- **Tip:** Use hydrating oils like coconut or olive oil to condition your hair. Regular oiling

and deep conditioning can address dryness and frizz.

7. Split Ends:
- **Tip:** Regularly trim your hair to prevent and manage split ends. Additionally, apply herbal hair masks with ingredients like Aloe Vera and hibiscus to strengthen and nourish your hair.

8. Hair Luster and Shine:
- **Tip:** Consider using Hibiscus and Aloe Vera-based products to add shine and luster to your hair. These natural ingredients enhance hair texture and appearance.

Remember that Ayurvedic remedies often require consistency and patience. The effectiveness of these tips may vary from person to person, so it's essential to find the practices and ingredients that work best for your unique hair condition. Consulting with an Ayurvedic practitioner can also provide personalized guidance tailored to your specific needs.

7.1 Dandruff and Itchy Scalp

Dandruff and an itchy scalp are common hair and scalp concerns that can be effectively addressed using Ayurvedic remedies. Here are Ayurvedic tips for managing dandruff and an itchy scalp:

1. Neem-Based Shampoo:
- **Tip:** Use a Neem-based shampoo. Neem has antifungal and antibacterial properties that can help combat dandruff and soothe an itchy scalp.

2. Aloe Vera Gel:

- **Tip:** Apply fresh aloe vera gel directly to your scalp. Aloe vera's cooling and moisturizing properties can alleviate itching and reduce dandruff.

3. Lemon Juice:
- **Tip:** Mix fresh lemon juice with water and apply it to your scalp. Lemon's acidity helps balance the pH of the scalp and control dandruff.

4. Fenugreek (Methi) Seeds:
- **Tip:** Soak fenugreek seeds overnight, grind them into a paste, and apply it to your scalp. Leave it on for about 30 minutes before rinsing. Fenugreek has antifungal properties and can reduce dandruff.

5. Coconut Oil and Camphor:

- **Tip:** Mix a small amount of camphor with coconut oil and apply it to your scalp. This can provide relief from itching and help control dandruff.

6. Hibiscus:
- **Tip:** Use hibiscus flower or leaf pastes on your scalp. Hibiscus helps soothe the scalp, reduce dandruff, and strengthen hair.

7. Avoid Harsh Chemicals:
- **Tip:** Avoid shampoos and hair products that contain harsh chemicals, as they can exacerbate scalp issues. Opt for natural, Ayurvedic products or homemade remedies.

8. Scalp Massage:
- **Tip:** Regular scalp massages with Ayurvedic hair oils, such as Neem or Amla oil,

can improve blood circulation, reduce itching, and nourish the scalp.

9. Ayurvedic Dietary Guidelines:
- **Tip:** Follow Ayurvedic dietary principles that are suitable for your dosha type. A balanced diet can contribute to overall scalp health.

Remember to be consistent with your chosen remedies, and it may take some time to see significant improvement. If dandruff and itching persist, it's advisable to consult with an Ayurvedic practitioner who can provide personalized guidance and recommendations tailored to your specific condition.

7.2 Premature Graying of Hair

Premature graying of hair is a common concern, and Ayurveda offers natural remedies to help manage and delay the graying process. Here are Ayurvedic tips for addressing premature graying of hair:

1. Amla (Indian Gooseberry):
- **Tip:** Incorporate Amla into your diet or hair care routine. Amla is a rich source of antioxidants and vitamin C, which can help slow down the graying process.

2. Amla Oil and Hair Masks:
- **Tip:** Use Amla oil or apply Amla-based hair masks to nourish your hair and scalp. These treatments can restore pigment and maintain your natural hair color.

3. Curry Leaves:
- **Tip:** Include curry leaves in your diet or make a paste with curry leaves and apply it to your hair. Curry leaves are rich in vitamins and

antioxidants that can help prevent premature graying.

4. Sesame Oil:
- **Tip:** Regularly massage your scalp with sesame oil. Sesame oil is known in Ayurveda for its anti-aging properties and can help prevent premature graying.

5. Yogurt and Fenugreek (Methi) Mask:
- **Tip:** Mix yogurt with ground fenugreek seeds and apply the paste to your hair. Fenugreek is believed to help maintain natural hair color.

6. Shikakai and Reetha (Soapnut):
- **Tip:** Use Shikakai and Reetha (Soapnut) as natural hair cleansers. These ingredients are gentle on the hair and can help maintain hair color.

7. Avoid Excessive Heat Styling:
- **Tip:** Excessive use of heat styling tools can contribute to premature graying. Limit the use of such tools and embrace your hair's natural texture.

8. Balanced Diet:
- **Tip:** Follow Ayurvedic dietary guidelines that align with your dosha type. A balanced diet with adequate vitamins and minerals is essential for hair health.

9. Stress Reduction:
- **Tip:** Incorporate stress-reduction techniques, such as yoga and meditation, into your daily routine. High stress levels can accelerate premature graying.

It's important to remember that Ayurvedic remedies often require consistency and patience. While these tips can help manage premature graying, results may vary from person to person. If you have concerns about premature graying, it's advisable to consult with an Ayurvedic practitioner or healthcare professional for personalized guidance and treatment options.

Chapter 8
Balancing Your Doshas for Healthy Hair

Balancing your doshas is a fundamental concept in Ayurveda for maintaining healthy hair and overall well-being. Here are some tips on how to balance your doshas for healthy hair:

1. Determine Your Dominant Dosha:
- Start by identifying your dominant dosha (Vata, Pitta, or Kapha) through an Ayurvedic assessment or consultation with an Ayurvedic practitioner.

2. Follow a Dosha-Specific Diet:
- Once you know your dominant dosha, tailor your diet to balance it. For example:
- If you're Vata-dominant, focus on warming, nourishing foods to prevent dryness.
- If you're Pitta-dominant, opt for cooling foods to avoid excess heat.
- If you're Kapha-dominant, prioritize lighter, warming foods to counter heaviness.

3. Ayurvedic Hair Oils:
- Choose hair oils that correspond to your dosha. For example:
- Vata types may benefit from sesame oil.
- Pitta types can use coconut or sunflower oil.
- Kapha types may prefer almond or mustard oil.

4. Lifestyle Practices:
- Align your lifestyle practices with your dosha:
- Vata types should maintain a regular routine to prevent anxiety and stress.
- Pitta types should practice cooling techniques like meditation to reduce excess heat.
- Kapha types should engage in regular exercise to prevent stagnation.

5. Herbal Hair Care:

- Select herbal products that are suitable for your dosha type. For example, Vata types may use hydrating herbs, while Pitta types can opt for cooling and soothing herbs.

6. Stress Reduction:
- Manage stress through practices like yoga and meditation, as stress can aggravate imbalances in your dosha.

7. Regular Scalp Massage:
- Incorporate regular scalp massages with dosha-specific oils to nourish the scalp and hair.

8. Monitor Seasonal Changes:
- Adjust your hair care routine based on the season. Ayurveda recognizes the impact of seasons on dosha balance and hair health.

9. Regular Exercise:

- Engage in regular physical activity to maintain a healthy metabolism and balance your doshas.

10. Consult an Ayurvedic Practitioner:
- For personalized guidance on balancing your doshas and maintaining healthy hair, consider consulting with an Ayurvedic practitioner who can provide tailored recommendations.

Balancing your doshas is an integral part of Ayurvedic hair care. By understanding your unique constitution and making adjustments in your diet, lifestyle, and hair care routine, you can promote healthy, vibrant hair and overall well-being.

8.1 Dosha-Specific Hair Care Recommendations

Here are dosha-specific hair care recommendations based on Ayurvedic principles:

Vata Dosha:
- Vata individuals often have dry and frizzy hair. To balance Vata dosha, consider the following:
  - **Hair Oil:** Use warm, nourishing oils like sesame oil or almond oil for regular scalp massages to prevent dryness.
  - **Shampoo:** Choose mild, hydrating shampoos that won't strip your hair of natural oils.
  - **Diet:** Include warm, grounding foods such as whole grains, nuts, and seeds in your diet. Hydrate well to combat dryness.
  - **Lifestyle:** Maintain a regular routine, get sufficient rest, and practice stress-reduction techniques like yoga and meditation.

Pitta Dosha:
- Pitta individuals may have fine hair and are prone to early graying. To balance Pitta dosha:
  - **Hair Oil:** Use cooling oils like coconut or sunflower oil for scalp massages to prevent excess heat.
  - **Shampoo:** Opt for mild, cooling shampoos that soothe the scalp.
  - **Diet:** Consume cooling foods like leafy greens, cucumbers, and coconut. Limit spicy and fried foods.
  - **Lifestyle:** Engage in stress-reduction practices to avoid excess heat buildup. Avoid overexposure to the sun.

Kapha Dosha:
- Kapha individuals may have thick, oily hair and are prone to dandruff. To balance Kapha dosha:

- **Hair Oil:** Use lighter oils like mustard or jojoba oil for scalp massages to prevent oiliness.
- **Shampoo:** Choose clarifying shampoos with herbal ingredients like Neem to manage oil and dandruff.
- **Diet:** Consume warming and light foods, including spices like ginger and black pepper. Avoid excessive sweets and heavy, fried foods.
- **Lifestyle:** Stay active and engage in regular exercise to prevent stagnation. Avoid oversleeping and maintain a dynamic routine.

These recommendations are general guidelines for dosha-specific hair care. Keep in mind that Ayurveda emphasizes personalized care. It's beneficial to consult with an Ayurvedic practitioner who can provide tailored advice based on your unique constitution and hair needs. Additionally, consider your specific hair concerns, such as dandruff, premature graying, or hair loss, and choose herbal remedies accordingly.

Chapter 9
Consultation with an Ayurvedic Practitioner

Consulting with an Ayurvedic practitioner can be highly beneficial for personalized guidance on various aspects of your health, including hair care. Here's what you can expect during a consultation with an Ayurvedic practitioner:

1. **Assessment of Your Dosha:** The practitioner will assess your unique constitution (Prakriti) and any current imbalances (Vikriti) by asking questions about your physical and mental characteristics, lifestyle, and health history.

2. **Detailed Discussion:** You'll have a thorough discussion about your hair concerns, such as hair type, hair loss, premature graying, dandruff, and any other issues you're experiencing.

3. **Diet and Lifestyle Recommendations:** The Ayurvedic practitioner will provide personalized recommendations for your diet

and lifestyle based on your dosha and hair concerns. This may include dietary adjustments, specific herbs or supplements, and daily routines.

4. **Herbal Remedies:** Depending on your concerns, the practitioner may suggest specific Ayurvedic herbal treatments, oils, shampoos, or masks to address your hair and scalp issues.

5. **Stress Reduction Techniques:** Ayurveda places a significant emphasis on stress reduction. You may receive guidance on practices like yoga, meditation, and breathing exercises to manage stress, which can impact your hair health.

6. **Follow-Up:** Typically, Ayurvedic consultations involve follow-up appointments to monitor progress and make any necessary adjustments to your treatment plan.

7. **Holistic Approach:** Ayurvedic practitioners consider your overall well-being, so they'll focus on not only hair care but also your general health and balance of your doshas.

8. **Duration and Cost:** The duration and cost of a consultation can vary depending on the practitioner, the complexity of your concerns, and the number of follow-up appointments required.

When seeking an Ayurvedic practitioner, look for someone with the appropriate credentials, training, and experience. Many Ayurvedic practitioners offer remote consultations if you don't have access to one locally. It's important to provide the practitioner with complete and honest information to receive the best recommendations for your specific needs.

Ayurvedic consultations can be a valuable step toward improving your hair health and overall well-being.

9.1 Finding the Right Ayurvedic Expert

Finding the right Ayurvedic expert is crucial for receiving personalized guidance and treatments for your health and well-being, including your hair care concerns. Here are some steps to help you find a qualified Ayurvedic practitioner:

1. Verify Qualifications:
   - Check the practitioner's qualifications and certifications. Look for a practitioner who has completed formal training in Ayurveda from a reputable institution.

2. Seek Recommendations:

- Ask for recommendations from friends, family, or healthcare professionals who may have experience with Ayurvedic practitioners.

3. Online Research:
   - Conduct online research to find Ayurvedic practitioners in your area or those who offer remote consultations. Review their websites and read client testimonials or reviews, if available.

4. Professional Associations:
   - Look for practitioners who are members of recognized Ayurvedic professional associations, such as the National Ayurvedic Medical Association (NAMA) in the United States.

5. Consult Multiple Practitioners:
   - Don't hesitate to schedule initial consultations with multiple practitioners to get a sense of their approach, communication style,

and whether you feel comfortable working with them.

6. Ask Questions:
   - During the consultation, ask the practitioner about their experience, treatment approach, and how they tailor recommendations to individual needs.

7. Treatment Specialization:
   - Consider whether the practitioner specializes in the specific areas of concern, such as dermatology, hair care, or other health issues.

8. Communication and Comfort:
   - Ensure that you feel comfortable communicating with the practitioner and that they listen to your concerns and provide clear, understandable guidance.

9. Transparency and Ethics:
   - Ensure that the practitioner is transparent about their treatment plans, fees, and any potential side effects or risks associated with Ayurvedic remedies.

10. Check for Licensure:
   - In some regions, Ayurvedic practitioners may need to be licensed or registered. Verify if this is required in your area.

11. Seek a Second Opinion:
   - If you have doubts or are unsure about a practitioner's recommendations, consider seeking a second opinion from another Ayurvedic expert.

Remember that Ayurveda is a holistic system of medicine, so the practitioner should consider your overall well-being in addition to your specific concerns. Your choice of an Ayurvedic expert should align with your individual health goals and preferences. Taking the time to find the right practitioner can lead to a more effective and personalized Ayurvedic treatment plan for your hair and overall health.

Chapter 10
Frequently Asked Questions

Here are some frequently asked questions (FAQs) related to Ayurvedic hair care:

1. What is Ayurvedic hair care?
- Ayurvedic hair care is a holistic approach to maintaining healthy hair using principles from Ayurveda, an ancient system of medicine from India. It involves using natural remedies, herbal treatments, and dietary changes to promote strong, shiny, and vibrant hair.

2. How can I determine my dosha type?
- Your dosha type (Vata, Pitta, or Kapha) can be determined through an Ayurvedic assessment, which considers your physical and mental characteristics, lifestyle, and health history. Ayurvedic practitioners can help identify your dominant dosha.

3. Which herbs are commonly used in Ayurvedic hair care?
- Common Ayurvedic herbs for hair care include Amla (Indian Gooseberry), Bhringraj, Neem, Shikakai, Reetha (Soapnut), Hibiscus, and Fenugreek, among others. These herbs offer various benefits for hair and scalp health.

4. Can Ayurveda help with hair growth?
- Yes, Ayurveda provides natural remedies and practices to promote hair growth. Herbs like Bhringraj and Amla are known for their hair-strengthening and growth-promoting properties.

5. How can I use Ayurvedic oils for hair care?
- Ayurvedic oils can be used for scalp massages or as pre-shampoo treatments. Apply the oil to your scalp and hair, leave it on for a period

(usually 30 minutes to an hour), and then wash your hair with a mild Ayurvedic shampoo.

6. Are there specific dietary guidelines in Ayurveda for healthy hair?
- Ayurveda emphasizes a balanced diet that aligns with your dosha type. Generally, it recommends eating fresh, whole foods, avoiding processed foods, and staying hydrated.

7. Can Ayurveda help with dandruff and itchy scalp?
- Yes, Ayurvedic remedies, such as Neem-based products and herbal rinses, can effectively address dandruff and soothe an itchy scalp.

8. How can Ayurveda help with premature graying of hair?
- Ayurveda offers remedies like Amla-based treatments and dietary adjustments to help

delay premature graying and maintain natural hair color.

9. What are some stress reduction techniques in Ayurveda for hair care?
- Ayurvedic stress reduction techniques include yoga, meditation, deep breathing exercises, and a balanced daily routine to manage stress, which can impact hair health.

10. How long does it take to see results with Ayurvedic hair care?
- The time it takes to see results varies depending on individual factors and concerns. Generally, consistency is key, and results may take several weeks to months to become noticeable.

These are some common FAQs related to Ayurvedic hair care. If you have specific questions or concerns, consulting with an Ayurvedic practitioner can provide personalized guidance and answers to your unique needs.

10.1 Common Queries About Ayurvedic Hair Care

Here are common queries and their answers related to Ayurvedic hair care:

1. Is Ayurvedic hair care safe for all hair types?
- Ayurvedic hair care is generally safe for all hair types. However, it's essential to choose products and remedies that are suitable for your specific hair concerns and dosha type.

2. Can Ayurveda cure hair loss?
- Ayurveda can help prevent and manage hair loss by addressing underlying imbalances and

promoting scalp and hair health. While it may not work for all cases, it can be effective for many individuals.

3. Can I use Ayurvedic hair care alongside other hair products?
- Yes, you can incorporate Ayurvedic hair care products and practices into your existing hair care routine. Just be mindful of any potential interactions with other products.

4. Are there any side effects of Ayurvedic hair care?
- Ayurvedic remedies are generally safe when used correctly. However, it's essential to do a patch test to ensure you are not allergic or sensitive to any ingredients.

5. How often should I do Ayurvedic hair treatments?

- The frequency of Ayurvedic hair treatments
depends on your specific concerns and the
recommendations of an Ayurvedic practitioner.
Generally, once a week or as needed is common
for treatments like oiling or masks.

6. Can Ayurveda help with thinning hair?
- Yes, Ayurveda can help with thinning hair by
promoting hair growth and strengthening the
hair. Herbs like Bhringraj and Amla are
beneficial for this concern.

**7. What is the best way to choose Ayurvedic
hair products?**
- To choose the best Ayurvedic hair products,
consider your dosha type and specific hair
concerns. Look for products that are free from
harsh chemicals and contain natural ingredients.

8. How long does it take to see results with Ayurvedic hair care?
- The time it takes to see results can vary from person to person and depends on the specific concern. Generally, consistency is key, and results may take several weeks to months to become noticeable.

9. Can Ayurveda help with hereditary hair issues?
- Ayurveda can help improve the health and condition of your hair, but its effectiveness in addressing hereditary hair issues may vary. It's best to consult with an Ayurvedic practitioner for guidance.

10. Is it necessary to consult an Ayurvedic practitioner for hair care?
- While not always necessary, consulting with an Ayurvedic practitioner can provide

personalized recommendations that are tailored to your unique constitution and hair concerns. It can be especially beneficial for complex or persistent issues.

These answers should help address some of the common queries about Ayurvedic hair care. Remember that Ayurvedic practices often require consistency and patience, and individual results may vary.

Chapter 11
Conclusion and Future Hair Care

In conclusion, Ayurvedic hair care offers a holistic and natural approach to maintaining healthy and vibrant hair. By understanding your dosha type, following dietary guidelines, incorporating herbal remedies, and adopting Ayurvedic lifestyle practices, you can promote strong, shiny, and well-nourished hair.

The future of hair care may increasingly include Ayurvedic principles as people seek more natural and sustainable alternatives to chemical-laden products. Ayurveda's focus on personalized care and overall well-being aligns with the growing trend of holistic and preventive health practices.

As you continue your Ayurvedic hair care journey, remember that consistency is key, and results may take time to become noticeable. Consulting with an Ayurvedic practitioner can provide tailored guidance for your specific needs and concerns.

Embracing Ayurvedic practices in your hair care routine not only helps maintain beautiful hair but also contributes to your overall health and well-being. Here's to healthy, lustrous, and naturally radiant hair in the future!

11.1 Summing up the Benefits of Ayurveda

let's sum up the benefits of Ayurveda:

1. **Holistic Well-Being:** Ayurveda is a holistic system that considers the well-being of the whole person, addressing physical, mental, and emotional health.

2. **Personalized Care:** Ayurveda provides individualized recommendations based on your unique constitution (dosha) and specific health concerns.

3. **Natural Remedies:** Ayurveda relies on natural ingredients and herbal remedies to promote health and treat various conditions, minimizing the use of chemicals.

4. **Preventive Approach:** Ayurveda emphasizes prevention through lifestyle, diet, and stress management, helping to maintain overall health and balance.

5. **Long-Term Health:** Ayurvedic practices aim to address root causes, leading to sustainable, long-term health benefits.

6. **Minimal Side Effects:** Ayurvedic treatments generally have minimal side effects when used correctly, making them suitable for many individuals.

7. **Promotion of Balance:** Ayurveda seeks to balance the doshas and promote harmony within the body, leading to improved health and well-being.

8. **Stress Reduction:** Ayurveda incorporates stress reduction techniques like yoga and meditation, which have a positive impact on mental and emotional health.

9. **Cultural Heritage:** Ayurveda is deeply rooted in Indian culture and has been practiced for thousands of years, offering a rich tradition of wellness.

10. **Complementary Medicine:** Ayurveda can complement conventional medicine, offering an integrative approach to health and well-being.

By embracing Ayurveda, individuals can experience these benefits and work towards achieving a state of balance and optimal health in a natural and holistic way.

11.2 Maintaining Healthy Hair with Ayurvedic Principles

Maintaining healthy hair with Ayurvedic principles involves a holistic approach that considers your dosha type, dietary habits, lifestyle, and the use of natural remedies. Here are some key practices to help you maintain healthy hair the Ayurvedic way:

1. Determine Your Dosha: Understand your dosha type (Vata, Pitta, or Kapha) to tailor your hair care routine and dietary choices to your specific needs.

2. Balanced Diet: Follow Ayurvedic dietary guidelines that align with your dosha type. Consume fresh, whole foods, and stay hydrated. Incorporate hair-healthy foods like Amla, coconut, and seeds.

3. Herbal Hair Care: Use Ayurvedic herbal hair products like shampoos, conditioners, and hair oils that are suitable for your dosha and hair type. Look for ingredients such as Amla, Bhringraj, Neem, Shikakai, and Hibiscus.

4. Scalp Massage: Regularly massage your scalp with Ayurvedic hair oils, such as coconut, sesame, or Amla oil. This stimulates blood circulation, nourishes the hair follicles, and promotes hair growth.

5. Herbal Hair Masks: Apply Ayurvedic hair masks with ingredients like yogurt, Fenugreek (Methi), and Aloe Vera to strengthen and condition your hair. Choose ingredients that match your dosha.

6. Stress Reduction: Incorporate stress-reduction techniques such as yoga and meditation into your daily routine. Stress can negatively impact your hair health, and these practices help maintain balance.

7. Seasonal Adaptations: Adjust your hair care routine based on the seasons and how they affect your dosha balance. For example, in hot weather, use cooling products to balance excess Pitta.

8. Lifestyle Practices: Maintain a regular daily routine to provide structure and stability, which is particularly important for Vata types. Balance your activities to avoid excessive stress or lethargy.

9. Dietary Supplements: Consider Ayurvedic dietary supplements or herbal formulations prescribed by an Ayurvedic practitioner if you have specific hair concerns.

10. Regular Trims: Trim your hair regularly to prevent split ends and maintain overall hair health.

By incorporating these Ayurvedic principles into your hair care routine, you can support the health and vibrancy of your hair, while also promoting overall well-being in a natural and holistic manner. Remember that consistency and patience are essential for lasting results.